Eye C

Revolutionary Guide to Natural Healing &
Solution to Problems Preventing a Clear Eye
Vision (Causes, Types, Prevention, Treatment,
Interraction & Diagnoses)

GRACE J. ALLEN

Table of Contents

Introduction

The eye is an organ that reacts to light and allows vision; the cells in the retina that allows mindful light belief are, which also enables eyesight, including color differentiation and the understanding of depth. The eye can differentiate between about 10 million colors and has the capacity to detect an individual photon.

This book is aimed at providing natural solution to eye problems. In this book; you would learn the fundamental causes of eye problems, eye infections and its symptoms and subsequently its treatment.

Also; you would learn the top factors that contribute to eye problems, such as red spot of the eye, eye twitch, vision problems and diabetes, cataracts, glaucomaretinopathy and freckles. You would likewise learn more about vision terms.

Like the eye of other mammals, the human being eyes non-image-forming photosensitive ganglion cells in the retina receive light indicators which affect modification of how big is the pupil, regulation, and suppression of the hormone melatonin and entrainment of your body clock.

After reading this book, I believe you would be glad you have read.

Structure

Blood vessels are seen within the sclera, and a strong limbal band round the iris.

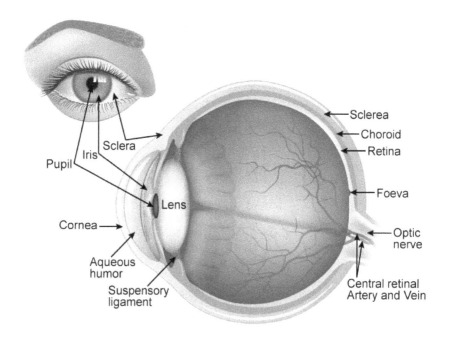

The outer elements of the eye:

The vision is made up of the anterior segment and the posterior segment; it's not shaped just like a perfect sphere. The anterior section comprises of the ***cornea, iris, and zoom lens***.

The cornea is clear and more curved, and it is from the bigger posterior portion, made up of the *vitreous, retina, choroid, and the external white shell called the sclera.* The cornea is normally about 11.5 mm (0.3 in) in diameter, and 0.5 mm (500 μm) thick near its center, the posterior chamber constitutes the rest of the five-sixths; its diameter is normally about 24 mm. The cornea and sclera are linked by a location termed the ***limbus***.

Iris is the pigmented round structure concentrically encircling the guts of the vision, the pupil, which is apparently black. The size of the pupil determines the quantity of light getting into the vision, which is modified by the iris' dilator and sphincter muscles.

Zoom lens - Light energy enters the vision through the cornea, through the pupil and then through the zoom lens; the lens form is transformed far near focus (accommodation), and it is managed by the ciliary muscle. Photons of light dropping on the light-sensitive cells of the retina (photoreceptor cones and rods) are changed into electric indicators that are sent to the mind by the optic nerve and interpreted as view and vision.

Chapter 1

Vision Floaters: Causes, Symptoms, and Treatment

Vision floaters appear as small pieces that drift through your field of eyesight. They could stand out when you have a look at something bright, just like a white paper or a blue sky. They could annoy you; however, they shouldn't hinder your sight.

When you yourself have a large floater, it could result in a solid hook shadow over your eyesight; but this may happen just using types of light. You are able to work out how to live with floaters and ignore them. You may see them less after some time. Just seldom do they get bad enough to require treatment.

What exactly are the symptoms?

Floaters earn their name by activity within your eyesight.

They have a tendency to dart away when you try to focus on them.

They can be found in many different shapes:

- Black or grey dots.

- Squiggly lines.

- Threadlike strands, which might be knobby and almost see-through.

- Cobwebs.

- Rings

Once you've them, they often times don't disappear completely. Nevertheless, you usually notice them less after a while.

WHAT CAN CAUSE Them?

Most floaters are small flecks from the proteins called collagen. They're area of the gel-like substance in the trunk of the eyes called the vitreous.

As you age, the protein fibers define the vitreous shrink because of little shreds that clump collectively. The shadows they cast on your own retina are floaters; in the event that you discover an adobe flash, it's as the vitreous offers drawn from your retina. If the floaters are new or significantly transformed or you abruptly begin to find flashes, watch your vision doctor ASAP.

These changes may appear at any age, but usually occur between 50 and 75. You're more likely to maintain these exact things if you're near-sighted or experienced cataract surgery.

It's uncommon, but floaters may also be based on:

· Eye disease.

· Eye injury.

· Diabetic retinopathy.

· Crystal-like dust that forms in the vitreous.

· Eye tumors

Serious eye disorders connected with floaters include:

· Detached retina.

· Torn retina.

· Bleeding inside your vitreous.

· Swollen vitreous or retina triggered by infections or an auto-immune condition.

· Eye tumors

What might resemble a floater may be the visual aura that is included with migraine headaches; it might look like what it really is when you put your vision to a kaleidoscope (it might actually move). It's different than the floaters and flashbulb type "flashes" including additional eyesight problems. It usually continues minutes and may involve the eyesight in both eyes. Nonetheless it completely resolves unless you possess another show.

When to start out to see the Doctor

In the event that you have several eyes floaters that doesn't change after a while, don't sweat it.

Go to the doctor ASAP in the event that you visit:

·	A sudden increase in the amount of floaters.

·	Flashes of light.

·	A lack of aspect vision.

·	Changes that can come on promptly and worsen as time passes.

·	Floaters after vision surgery or vision trauma.

Eye pain

Choose a doctor that has encounter with retina problems. In the event that you don't get support immediately, you could lose your view.

How Are Floaters Treated?

Benign ones seldom require treatment; if certainly they annoy you, try to keep these things out of the field of eyesight. Move your eye; this shifts the liquid around.

When you yourself have a lot of that they end your eyesight, your eyesight doctor may suggest surgery called a vitrectomy; he'll get rid of the vitreous and replace it having a sodium solution.

You've got complications like:

· Detached retina.

· Torn retina

Cataracts: The opportunity is low, but if these problems happen, they are able to permanently harm your vision.

Chapter 2

Eye Pain: What are the causes?

Everybody will establish sore eyes eventually; sometimes, they progress independently, however they can also be an indicator of something a lot more serious. Your eye doctor will get out what's happening and find out the proper treatment for you personally.

Where does it hurt?

Sometimes pain results from a problem within your eyesight or the parts around it, such as for example:

· Cornea: The obvious windows in leading of the eyes that concentrate light.

· Sclera: The whites of the eyes.

· Conjunctiva: The ultra-thin covering of the sclera as well as the within of the eyelid.

· Iris: The colored part of your vision, using the

pupil in the guts.

· Orbit: A bony cave (vision socket) inside your skull where in fact the eye and its own muscles are available.

· Extraocular muscles: They rotate your eyesight.

· Nerves: They carry visual info from your own eye towards the human brain.

· Eyelids: Outdoors coverings that protect and spread dampness over your eye.

Common Eyesight Problems

· Blepharitis: An swelling or infections from the eyelid which typically isn't painful

· Conjunctivitis (pink eye): That's irritation from the conjunctiva. Maybe it's from allergic reactions or attacks (viral or bacterial). Arteries in the conjunctiva swell. It creates the part of your eyes that's usually white look red. Your vision may well also get itchy and gunky. This issue usually isn't painful.

· Corneal abrasions: That's the state name for any scratch upon this portion of your vision. It sounds minimal, nonetheless it could harm. It's easy to accomplish, too. It is possible to scratch your eyesight while massaging it. A medical doctor offers you antibiotic drops. It'll progress in just a few days without further problems.

· Corneal infections (keratitis): A swollen or contaminated cornea can also be the effect of the bacterial or viral infection. You may be more likely to acquire it in the event that you leave your connections in overnight or wear filthy lenses.

· International bodies: Something within your eye, just like a little of dirt and grime, can irritate it. Try to wash it out with artificial tears or normal water. In the event that you don't obtain it out, it could scrape your eye.

· Glaucoma: This group of circumstances causes liquid to build up inside your eyes, which places pressure on your own optic nerve. In the event that you don't treat it, you could drop your view. Generally, you will find no early symptoms. But a sort called severe angle-closure glaucoma; causes pressure inside your vision to go up suddenly. Symptoms include severe vision pain, nausea, headaches, and worsening eyesight. It really is an unexpected emergency. You'll need treatment ASAP in order to avoid blindness.

· Uveitis: A swelling within your eyesight from trauma, attacks, or problems with your immune system. Symptoms include pain, red eyes, and, often, worse eyesight.

· Optic neuritis: An inflammation from the nerve that travels from your trunk from the eyeball in to the mind. Multiple sclerosis and other conditions or attacks tend to be at fault. Medical indications include insufficient eyesight and sometimes deep distress when you look laterally.

· Sinusitis: Contamination in one of your sinuses. When pressure accumulates behind your eye, it could stress using one or both edges.

· Stye: That is clearly a sensitive bump on the

benefit of your eyelid; it happens when an important oil gland, eyelash, or locks follicle gets contaminated or inflamed. You may hear a medical doctor call it a chalazion or hordeolum.

Other Symptoms

Eye pain may appear alone or with additional symptoms, like:

·   Less vision.

·   Discharge (Maybe it's very clear or solid and colored)

·   Foreign body sensation (the feeling that something is usually in the vision, whether real or imagined)

·   Headache.

·   Light sensitivity.

·   Nausea/vomiting.

·   Red-eye or pink eye .

·   Tearing

Your eye is crusted shut with discharge when you awaken. Additional symptoms, plus a sore eye, can be viewed as a clue from what's resulting in the pain.

Assessments to Diagnose Eyes Pain

Discover your eyes doctor when you have eye pain, especially if you possess less vision, headache, or nausea.

Vision doctors use some tools to diagnose vision pain:

· A slit-lamp exam uses shiny light to look at all of the constructions of the vision.

· Dilating drops boost your pupil to permit doctor to find out deep in to the eye.

· A tonometer can be an instrument that measures eyesight pressure. The physician uses it to diagnose glaucoma.

Treatments

Exactly like causes varies, so do treatments. They concentrate on the specific cause of eye pain.

- Conjunctivitis: Antibacterial eye drop can cure bacterial conjunctivitis. Antihistamines through eyes drop, a tablet or syrup can improve conjunctivitis from allergic reactions.

- Corneal abrasions: These heal independently as time passes. A medical doctor might recommend an antibiotic ointment or drops.

- Glaucoma: You'll obtain eyes drop as well as perhaps pills to reduce pressure. If certainly, they don't really work, you may want surgery.

- Infected cornea: You may want antiviral or antibacterial eye drop.

- Iritis: The physician will treat this with steroid, antibiotic, or antiviral eyes drop.

- Optic neuritis: It's treated with corticosteroids.

- Styes: Use warm compresses in the home for two days.

The only way to deal with the resources of eye pain and

to get the proper treatment is to see a doctor. Your eyesight is valuable; protect it by taking eye pain significantly.

Chapter 3

Eye Infections

In case your eyes are itchy and they're beginning to change colour of pink, you should be able to call a medical doctor immediately; however, there are key signs that may offer an accurate clues to just what is usually wrong.

Contamination within your eyes can get to many other ways. A good deal is dependent upon which a part of your vision has got the problem. For instance, you may get symptoms inside your;

·   Eyelid.

·   Cornea (a definite surface that addresses the surface of the vision).

·   Conjunctiva (a thin, moist area that addresses the within from the eyelids and external layer of the eyesight).

Symptoms of the attention Infection

It's likely you have symptoms in one or both eyes when you yourself have an infection. Think about this kind of trouble:

· Pain or discomfort.

· Itchy eyes.

· A sense that something's on or within your eye.

· Eye hurts if it's bright (light awareness).

· Burning up inside your eyes.

· Small, unpleasant lump under your eyelid or in the bottom of the eyelashes.

· Eyelid is usually sensitive when you touch it.

· Eye won't stop tearing up.

· Discomfort within your eyes.

How your eyes look. It's likely you have changes like:

- Discharge out of just one 1 or both eyes that's yellow, green, or clear.

- Red color in the "whites" of the eyes.

- Swollen, red, or crimson eyelids.

- Crusty lashes and lids, especially every day.

You will probably find you have blurry eyesight. Several other problems you'll find are fever, trouble wearing contacts, and swollen lymph nodes near your ear.

Types of Vision Infections

Once you observe your physician, you may hear him/her use medical ailments like:

Pinkeye (conjunctivitis): this is actually the contamination of the conjunctiva and usually provides your eye a red tint. Maybe it's the effect of the bacteria or trojan, although sometimes you'll find it from an allergic attack or irritants. It's common to get pinkeye when you yourself have a cold.

Keratitis: This is the contamination of the cornea. Maybe

it's due to bacteria, infections, or parasites in normal water; it's a common problem for those who wear contacts.

Stye: It might appear as unpleasant red bumps under your eyelid or in the bottom of the eyelashes. You keep these things when the fundamental oil glands inside your eyelid or eyelashes get infected with bacteria.

Fungal eyes infections: It's uncommon to get attacks from fungi; however, they could be severe in the event that you undertake. Many fungal vision attacks happen after a vision injury, especially if your vision was scraped with something from an herb, just like a stay or a thorn. You can also get one in the event that you wear contacts and don't clean them properly.

Uveitis: That's contamination of the guts degree of your eyesight, called the uvea. It's sometimes connected with an inflammatory disease like arthritis rheumatoid or lupus.

Before making a decision on the very best treatment for your infection, a medical doctor should have a look at your eye and may likewise have a tissue or fluid sample. She'll mail it to a laboratory, where it gets examined under a microscope or placed right into a dish to make a culture.

Predicated on the actual lab findings, a medical doctor may recommend medication you take orally, a cream you apply on your own eyelid and eyes, or eyes drop (if chlamydia); is due to an injury, allergy, irritant, or other health, she may suggest other treatments to handle those issues. You must not wear contacts until your eye infection has solved.

Why is there gunk in my own eye?

Have you any idea that you blink 10-20 occasions one minute? Every time it happens, your eyes get yourself a few milliseconds of safety and quick wetness shower. Blinking also washes away the mucus your eyes make all day every day.

You are unable to blink that gunk away if you are asleep, it just gathers in the part of your vision closest to your nasal (where your lashes meet your eyelid). The right name because of this is usually rheum; nevertheless, you almost certainly call it rest.

You may place cream-colored mucus occasionally, which can be normal; it forms when an irritant, like mud or dirt, gets within your vision. But eye release can sign something you can't blink or wipe away.

Pinkeye: Your eyelid is lined having a see-through membrane called the conjunctiva. Furthermore, it addresses the white portion of your eyeball. This coating is definitely filled up with tiny arteries you normally can't discover. If they get infected, the whites of the eye look red or pink, hence the name pinkeye. A medical doctor may well also call it conjunctivitis.

It's due to allergic reactions or a viral infection. Vision release is a common sign; babies can buy it if a rip duct hasn't exposed completely.

Clogged tear duct: You have a rip gland above each eyeball. They make the liquid that gets wiped across your eyesight when you blink. It drains into ducts in the part of your eyes closest to your nasal. If a rip leave duct is clogged, that liquid has nowhere to go to. The duct will get badly infected and cause release.

Dry vision: Tears are constructed of four things: normal water, oils, mucus, and antibodies. If their balance is off, or in case your rip glands stop making tears, your eye gets dry. Whenever your vision doesn't get enough liquid, it tells your anxious system to send some. That sometimes comes in to play the correct execution of crisis tears, which don't contain the same nourishing balance as regular tears. Crisis tears with an excessive amount of mucus can lead to strings of gunk in or around your eyesight.

Corneal ulcer: The cornea addresses your iris, the colored part of your eyes, plus your pupil, that allows the light in. It's uncommon, but an ulcer can occur when there are a vision contamination or extreme case of dry out vision; it might create discharge.

Chapter 4

What are Eye Freckles?

Maybe you've had slightly red color around your eye because you were a young child, or maybe you only discovered you feature a vision freckle within a checkup; a freckle within your vision may seem unusual, but they're common and usually safe.

When you yourself have one, your eyesight doctor might want to watch it after a while. It's rare; however, they are able to turn into some sort of malignancy called melanoma. So whether they're old or new, it's always best if you have them tested.

Exactly what are they?

Eyes Freckle: You will find two types of vision freckles; the foremost is theoretically referred to as a nevus; they're much like moles on your own skin layer. "Nevus" means "mole." Many of these nevi (the plural of nevus) are easy to recognize. But others are concealed in the trunk of the vision, where nobody however your eyesight doctor will ever see them; they have different titles based on where they might be:

· Conjunctival nevus: At the top of the eye.

· Iris nevus: In the colored part of your eye.

· Choroidal nevus: Under your retina (in the trunk of the eyes)

Nevi could be yellow, darkish, grey, or an assortment of colours, which are manufactured by special cells called melanocytes, which give your skin layer as well as your eye their color. Those cells are often disseminated, but if enough of the clump joins, they are kind nevus.

The other sort of eye freckles is named iris freckles; they may be small flecks in the shaded portion of your vision. They're like the freckles on your own skin layer than moles (they're just at the top of the vision and don't impact its shape); about half 50 % of most people have iris freckles. Some types of nevi form before delivery, while iris freckles will get to older adults.

Chapter 5

Glossary of Vision Terms

·   Achromatopsia: Inadequate certain receptors within your retinas. Your eyesight won't be razor-sharp, and you'll be almost or completely colourblind. It's an inherited condition.

·   Alpha-2 agonists: Medications used to deal with glaucoma. They support aqueous laughter drain out of the vision and prevent your vision from making more of it - the result: Lower pressure inside your eye.

·   Amblyopia: A problem also known as "lazy eyesight" that begins in child years. Because one or the other vision isn't used constantly to provide a razor-sharp image, eyesight doesn't develop precisely how it will. If it isn't treated, one vision will be weaker.

·   Aqueous humor: The clear, watery liquid between your lens and cornea.

· Astigmatism: Whenever your cornea is usually shaped much like a football in comparison with a baseball. It causes blurry eyesight. It is possible to right it with eye glasses, contacts, or surgery.

· Beta-blockers: Medicated vision drops that treat glaucoma. They cause your eyesight to makes less aqueous laughter, which decreases the pressure within it.

· Carbonic anhydrase inhibitors: Medications that treat glaucoma. They cause your eyes to create less aqueous laughter, which decreases pressure.

· Choroid: The coating of arteries between your retina and sclera.

· Choroiditis: Some sort of uveitis, or irritation from the uvea, the eye's middle level. It causes the coating beneath your retina to become inflamed.

· Conjunctiva: A thin degree of cells that lines the within of the eyelids as well as the outer regions of your sclera.

· Conjunctivitis: Swelling of the conjunctiva, also

called pinkeye.

· Cornea: The obvious front side outer coating of the vision; it addresses the iris.

· Cryotherapy: Surgery that freezes and destroys abnormal cells.

· Cyclitis: Some sort of uveitis that inflames the guts part of your vision. Additionally, it could impact the muscle that concentrates your contact lens. Cyclitis should come on instantly and last almost a year.

· Dilation: When the vision doctor gives you medicated drops to start your pupil.

· Enucleation: Whenever your vision is surgically removed.

· Hyperopia: When it's hard to find out items up close, but things farther away are clearer. The most common name as a result of this is farsightedness.

· Intraocular: Of or linked to the within of the eyesight.

· Iris: The colored membrane around your pupil. It expands and agrees to regulate the amount of light that enters your eyes.

· Iritis: The most typical type of uveitis. It impacts the iris, which is often connected with autoimmune circumstances like arthritis rheumatoid. It could arrive suddenly and may last up to eight weeks, despite having treatment.

· Legal blindness: Whenever your vision, in both eyes, can't be corrected or when you yourself have an obvious field of 20 levels or less. (Your vision doctor may call this tunnel eyesight.)

· Low vision: When you're either legally blind (you have an obvious acuity of less than 20/200 tunnel vision) or have visible acuity between 20/70 and 20/200, whatever the usage of glasses or contacts.

· Macula: The central portion of your retina, which is essential for high res eyesight. When it's healthy, you'll possess a definite, sharpened vision.

· Macular edema: A swelling from the macula which makes it hard to find out. It usually results from damage or disease.

· Myopia: If it's difficult to see items in the space while near items have emerged more clearly. Also called nearsightedness.

· Nighttime blindness: When you yourself have trouble viewing in dim or darkened circumstances. It could derive from inadequate supplement A. Less often; it's an indicator of retinitis pigmentosa.

· Nyctalopia: See nighttime blindness.

· Ocular: Of or linked to your vision.

· Ophthalmologist: Doctors who concentrate on the medical and medical procedures of the attention. They may be either doctor of medication (MD) or doctors of osteopathy (DO). They provide total eye treatment, like eyesight services, eye examinations, medical and health care, analysis and treatment of disease, and management of problems from other conditions, like diabetes.

· Ophthalmoscope: A drum that examines your retina. You'll find two types:

· Immediate: Examines the guts of the retina.

· Indirect: Checks your complete retina.

· Optic nerve: It bears light signs from your own retina towards the mind, which becomes images.

· Optometrist: Physician trained to examine, diagnose, treat, and manage eyesight diseases and disorders. They could prescribe eyeglasses and contacts aswell as check your eye's inner and external buildings for diseases such as for example glaucoma, retinal diseases, and cataracts, or common conditions like nearsightedness, farsightedness, astigmatism, and presbyopia. Generally, in most state they aren't permitted to do laser or additional eye surgeries.

· Peripheral vision: All you discover from the medial side of the eye, not your immediate kind of vision.

· Photocoagulation: Some sort of laser surgery used in order to avoid loss of blood or repair broken tissue. It's commonly used to deal with retinal circumstances like problems from diabetes. Furthermore, it can help treat vision tumors.

· Pinkeye: See conjunctivitis.

· Presbyopia: Whenever your eye can't change concentrate to find out items close up. It isn't a sickness, but a fundamental element of the eye's natural aging process. It impacts everyone eventually in life. It usually arises around this group 40 to 45.

· Pupil: The circular, dark central starting inside your vision. That is where the light comes into play.

· Refraction: Precisely how your eyesight bends light, so a graphic focuses on your retina. Also, the duty through which a medical doctor determines the optical prescription for contacts or glasses.

· Refractive error: Whenever your eyes don't bend light, precisely how it will. Images are out of concentrate. The most typical refractive mistakes are astigmatism, farsightedness, and nearsightedness. Your vision doctor can appropriate it with prescription eyeglasses, contacts, or occasionally, laser corrective surgery.

· Retina: The thin degree of nerves that lines the trunk of the vision. It senses light and indicates your optic nerve and brain to create images.

· Retinitis pigmentosa: A few of many retina conditions you are able to inherit; each enables you to lose sight after a while. Typically a decrease in eyesight may be the first indication accompanied from your eyesight tunneling because of just what is self-explanatory. Eventually, your central eyesight may decrease.

· Retinoblastoma: A malignant tumor that forms on your own retina. It frequently happens in children under age 5. It might impact one or both eyes.

· Sclera: The external coating from the eyeball that forms the whites of the eye.

· Strabismus: Whenever your eyes aren't aligned and can't point in the same path at the same time. The crossed eye is one sort of strabismus.

· Tunnel eyesight: Whenever your eyesight is entirely gone, conditions like retinitis pigmentosa and untreated glaucoma could cause tunnel eyesight.

· Visible acuity: How you observe as measured having a vision chart.

· Visual field: Your complete collection of view, including peripheral vision.

· Vitrectomy: With this surgical procedure, the vitreous laughter is removed from your eyeball and replaced using a definite sodium solution or temporarily having a gas bubble. It will help when marks or bleeding within your vitreous blocks your eyesight.

Vitreous humor: The very clear gel-like substance in the heart of the eyeball.

Chapter 6

Vision Problems & Diabetes

Like a diabetic patient, the capability to take safety precautions in reducing the risk of developing vision problems is vital because blindness is 20 occasions more frequent in individuals who have diabetes. The three major eye issues that people with diabetes need to be aware of are cataracts, glaucoma, and retinopathy.

In order to avoid vision problems, you should:

·   Control your blood sugar.

·   Have your eye checked one or more times a year by an ophthalmologist (eyes specialist).

·   Control high blood pressure and lipids.

Contact a medical doctor if the next happens:

·   Dark spots within your vision

·   Flashes of light.

Cataracts

A cataract is a clouding or fogging from the zoom lens in the vision. At this period, light cannot enter the vision and eyesight is impaired.

Symptoms

- Blurred vision

- Glared vision

- Treatment

Treatment - Surgery accompanied by glasses, contacts, or contact lens implant might help in intense situations such as this.

Glaucoma

Glaucoma can be an illness from the optic nerve (the "wire" that connects the vision to your brain and transmits light impulses to your brain). If the pressure in the vision accumulates, it could damage this optic nerve.

Often, you will find NO symptoms from glaucoma; the next symptoms might occur:

·   Loss of eyesight or visual field

·   Headaches

·   Eye pains (pain)

·   Halos around lights

·   Blurred vision

·   Watering eyes

Treatment

·   Special eye drops

·   Laser therapy

·   Medication

·   Surgery

Prevention - Have your eyes doctor display the state of eye for glaucoma annually.

Retinopathy

Problems with the retina are called diabetic retinopathy; this issue is usually developed consequently when liquid leaks from arteries in to the eyesight or abnormal arteries formed in the vision. If retinopathy isn't found early or isn't treated, blindness can happen.

Symptoms

Sometimes you can find no symptoms of retinopathy, but two common symptoms are:

· Blurred vision

· Places or lines inside your vision

Treatment

· Laser therapy

· Surgery

· Injections into eyes (advanced retinopathy)

Prevention

Possess your eyes doctor display the state of the eye around the screen for retinopathy annually.

Women with pre-existing diabetes who have a baby should have an intensive vision exam through the first trimester and close follow-up with a vision doctor during carrying a child, (This recommendation won't connect to women who develop gestational diabetes, because they are not in peril for retinopathy.)

Chapter 7

Top Factors behind Eye Problems

Lots of people possess eyesight problems at onetime or another. Some are small and can disappear independently (easy to deal with in the home), while some need a specialist's treatment. Whether your eyesight isn't what it utilized to exist, or never was that great, you will find actions you may take to really get your eyes health backwards on the right course.

Below are some typically common sight problems;

· Eyestrain

Anyone who reads forever, works together with a pc, or drives long distances is susceptible to this issue; it happens when you overuse your eye, they get exhausted and have to rest, the same as some other area of the body.

If the eyes feel strained, supply them with some time off. If they're nonetheless weary after a few days, check with your doctor to make sure it isn't another problem.

·   Red-Eyes

Your eyes look bloodshot. Why?

That is when the top of eye is protected in arteries that expand when the first is annoyed or infected, which in turn causes the red look.

Red-eye is truly a symptom of another eye condition, like conjunctivitis (pinkeye) or sun damage from not sporting shades as time passes. If over-the-counter vision drops and rest don't clear it up, see a medical doctor.

Eyestrain could possibly be the solution to the problem, therefore slight sleep during the night will do. If an injury's the reason, obtain it examined by a medical doctor.

·   Nighttime Blindness

That is a sight problem that means it is difficult for someone to see during the night, stick to course around any dark places. Nearsightedness, cataracts, keratoconus, and inadequate supplement A; all create a kind of evening blindness that doctors can fix.

A lot of people are born with this problem, or it might develop from a degenerative disease associated with the retina, which always can't end up being treated. When you yourself have it, you'll need to be spare careful in parts of low light.

- Lazy Eye

Sluggish eye, or amblyopia, happens when one eye doesn't develop properly; this happens when "this eye" vision is weak, and it'll move "lazily" around as the other eye remains put. It's been observed to occur mostly amidst babies, children, and adults, and seldom affects both eyes.

Treatment should be sought immediately for newborns and children; lifelong vision problems could be prevented if a sluggish eye is recognized and treated during early childhood. Treatment includes corrective contacts or glasses and employing a patch or different ways of creating a kind to utilize the sluggish eye.

- Cross Eye (Strabismus) and Nystagmus

If the eyes aren't prearranged with each other when you have a look at something, it's likely you have strabismus; that is also called crossed eye or walleye. This problem won't disappear completely if you don't obtain an ophthalmologist, or eyes specialist, to boost it.

You'll find so many treatments, including vision therapy, to create your eyes stronger. Surgery can be a choice. A medical doctor will test thoroughly your eye to find out which treatment my work right for you personally.

- Color blindness

When you can't see certain colors, or can't tell the difference between them (usually reds and greens), you may be colorblind; it happens when the colour cells within your vision (the physician will call them cone cells) are absent or don't work.

When it's most unfortunate, you can only see in tones of gray, but that is rare. Lots of people who've it receive delivery with it; nevertheless, you can buy it later in life from certain drugs and diseases. Men will be made up of it than women.

Your eye doctor can diagnose it with an easy test. There's no treatment if you're delivered with it, but special connections and eyeglasses might help many visitors to inform the difference between certain colors.

·   Uveitis

This is actually the name for a number of diseases that cause inflammation from the uvea (the guts layer from the vision which provides the most arteries).

These diseases can destroy eye tissue, as well as cause eye loss; symptoms may disappear completely quickly or last for an extended period. People with immune system circumstances like AIDS, arthritis rheumatoid, or ulcerative colitis could become much more likely to own uveitis. Symptoms range from:

·   Blurred vision

·   Eye pain

·   Eye redness

- Light sensitivity

See a medical doctor when you have these symptoms, and they also don't disappear completely in just a few days. There are various types of treatment for uveitis, with regards to the type you have.

- Presbyopia

This happens when you lose the energy, despite great way vision, to find out close objects. After age 40 roughly, it's likely you have to transport a book or other reading material further from your own eyes to create it better to read.

Reading glasses, contacts, LASIK, which is laser vision surgery, and other methods enable you to restore sound reading vision.

- Floaters

They may be tiny places or specks that float over the field of eyesight; lots of people detect them in well-lit rooms or outside on the bright day.

Floaters are often normal; however, they sometimes can be viewed as an indicator of a significant eyesight problem, like retinal detachment. That's when the retina behind your eyes separates from your coating underneath; you might discover light flashes combined with floaters or a dark shadow come across the benefit of your view.

If you see an abrupt change in the type of level of areas or flashes you observe or a brand new dark "drape" inside your peripheral eyesight, head to your vision doctor at the initial opportunity.

· Dry Eyes

This happens whenever the eyes can't make enough top quality tears. It could feel like something is usually within your vision, or like it's burning, extreme dryness can lead to some insufficient eyesight.

Some treatments include:

· Utilizing a humidifier in your own home

- Special eye drops that work like real tears

- Plugs inside your rip ducts to lessen drainage

- Lipiflow can be another treatment that serves as a surgical procedure that uses warmth and pressure to deal with dry eyes

- Testosterone eyelid cream

Supplements with fish oil and omega-3

If the dry eye problem is chronic, it's likely you have dry eye disease; your physician could prescribe medicated drops like cyclosporine (Cequa, Restasis) or lifitegrast (Xiidra) to stimulate rip production.

- Excess Tearing

It has nothing to do with your feelings; you might be delicate to light, wind flow, or heat changes. Try to protect your eye by shielding them or gaining sunglasses (choose wrap-around structures -- they stop more wind flow than additional styles).

Tearing may possibly also signal a more severe problem,

as vision contamination or a blocked rip duct. Your eyesight doctor can treat these conditions.

· Cataracts

These are cloudy areas that develop in the vision lens. A wholesome zoom lens is definitely clear like a camera's; light goes on through it to your retina (the trunk of the eyes where images are ready). When you yourself have a cataract, you can't find as well and may see glare or a halo around lamps during the night.

Cataracts often kind slowly; they don't really cause symptoms like pain, inflammation, or tearing in the vision. Some stay small and don't affect your view, if indeed they make improvement and impact your eyesight, surgery generally works to consider it back.

· Glaucoma

Your eye is comparable to a tire: Some pressure within it really is normal and safe, but levels that are an excessive amount may damage your optic nerve. Glaucoma may be the name for many diseases that cause this issue.

A common form may be the main start angle glaucoma; lots of people who've it don't experience early symptoms or pain, so that it is vital that you maintain together with your regular vision exams.

It doesn't happen often, but glaucoma could be due to:

· A personal problems for the vision

· Blocked arteries

· Inflammatory disorders from the vision

· Treatment includes prescription vision drops or surgery.

· Retinal Disorders

The retina is a thin coating around the trunk of the eye that comprises cells that gather images and pass these to the mind; retinal disorders stop this transfer. The retinal disorder varies in various types/conditions the following:

- Age-related macular degeneration identifies a break down of a small area of the retina called the macula.

- Diabetic retinopathy can be injury to the arteries within your retina due to diabetes.

- Retinal detachment happens when the retina separates through the layer underneath.

It's vital that you get early diagnosis and possess these circumstances treated.

· Conjunctivitis (Pinkeye)

In this issue, the tissue that lines the trunk of the eyelids and covering your sclera gets inflamed; it might cause redness, scratching, burning, tearing, release, or a feeling that something is certainly inside your eyesight.

Causes include illness, connection with chemicals and irritants, or allergic reactions. Wash the hands often to reduce your prospect of getting it.

· Corneal Diseases

The cornea may be the clear, dome-shaped "window" in the front end of the eye; it can benefit to focus on the light that can be found in. Disease, injury, and connection with toxins could cause this damage. Indicators include:

- Red eyes.

- Watery eyes.

- Pain.

- Reduced vision, or a halo effect

The main treatment plans include:

- A fresh eyeglasses or contacts prescription.

- Medicated eyes drop.

- Surgery

- Eyelid Problems

Your eyelids execute a good deal for you personally; they protect your eyes, spread tears over its surface, and limit the amount of light that may enter.

Pain, itching, tearing, and degree of sensitivity to light are normal symptoms of eyelid problems; you might feature blinking spasms or swollen outer sides near your eyelashes.

Treatment could include proper cleaning, medication, or surgery.

· Vision Changes

As you get older, you will probably find that you can't see aswell as you once did; that's normal (you'll probably need eyeglasses or contacts). You may choose to hold surgery (LASIK) to boost your vision, in the event that you already have eyeglasses; you may want a stronger prescription.

Anytime you come with an abrupt lack of eyesight, or everything appears blurry (even if it's short-term), see a doctor right away.

· Issues with contacts

They work nicely for some; nevertheless, you will need to provide for them, wash the hands before you touch them, and observe the procedure guideline that was incorporated with your prescription. Also, follow these guidelines:

- Never wet them by putting them in the jaws. That could make contamination much more likely.

- Ensure that your lenses fit properly, so they don't scrape your eyes.

- Use vision drops that say they're safe for contacts.

Never use homemade saline solutions, even though some lenses are FDA-approved for sleeping in them will not mean you must do it regularly, carrying this out raises the opportunity of significant infection.

In the event that you do everything ideal but still find yourself getting your connections, see your vision doctor. You likely have allergic reactions, dry eyes, or be better off with eyeglasses. Knowing the actual problem normally, you are able to decide what's best for you.

WHAT CAN CAUSE Eye Freckles?

Doctors don't know why a lot of people have them aswell as others don't, but something or two may impact your chances:

·   Competition: Choroidal nevi (in the trunk of the eyesight) certainly are many more common in white people or individuals who have lighter skin shades than in dark people.

·   Sun Exposure: It's possible that sun harm might boost your probability of nevi, and there's evidence that iris freckles are linked to being away in the sunlight. A 2017 research discovered that people who spent more time in sunlight experienced more iris freckles.

Do Eyes Freckles Need Treatment?

Usually, eye freckles are harmless, the same as most moles and freckles on your own skin layer; they're improbable to influence your eyesight or cause any problems. The only reason you might want treatment for an eye freckle is if a medical doctor thinks maybe it's a melanoma.

See A MEDICAL DOCTOR

If you've noticed a location or freckle inside your eyes, it's not likely a problem; but it's vital that you obtain it tested with a vision doctor (optometrist or an ophthalmologist).

During your appointment, a medical doctor might want to have an image from the freckle as well as perhaps do some imaging scans to check it out even more closely. You might return every half a year approximately to guarantee the freckle hasn't transformed (like growing bigger). If it nonetheless appears the same as time passes, you often will switch to annual checkups.

Other reasons to find out a vision doctor include:

·   A freckle within your eyesight that's grown or changed its form or color.

·   Eye pain.

·   You see blinking lights

Other changes inside your vision

To guard your eye, wear glasses that visit least 99% of Ultraviolet rays when you're outdoors. While we don't know for several, shades might lower the possibilities safe nevus can be melanoma. Plus, they definitely reduce your probability of obtaining cataracts and additional serious eye problems.

Chapter 8

Red Spot of the Eye

The red colorization around your eye might appear frightening, but it's usually no significant offer. There are many tiny arteries in the middle of your white of the eyesight as well as the sclera (the film that addresses it). Sometimes they break.

You do not even understand that you have a red spot (its standard name is sub-conjunctival hemorrhage) until you try looking inside a mirror; you won't notice any observable symptoms like eyesight changes, release, or pain. The only soreness it's likely you have is usually a scratchy sense at the top of the eyes.

THE CAUSES OF Them?

Most happen whenever your blood pressure spikes as a result to:

·   Strong sneezing.

- Straining.

- Powerful coughing.

- Vomiting

Some red spots are based on an injury or illness, like:

- Approximately rubbing your eye.

- Trauma, as being a foreign object stuck within your eye

Contact lenses

- Viral infection.

- Surgery.

Less common causes include:

- Diabetes.

- High blood pressure.

- Medicines that produce you bleeding easily (such as for example aspirin or bloodstream thinners like

Coumadin).

· Bloodstream clotting disorders.

How are they Diagnosed?

A medical doctor can inform you have a subconjunctival hemorrhage simply from looking at your eye.

How Are They Treated?

Most red spots heal independently without treatment; based on how big it really is, it could take a few days or a week or two to disappear completely. If it starts to feel annoying, it's Okay to use artificial tears.

CAN I Prevent Them?

If you wish to rub your vision, take action gently; if a red place keeps returning, a medical doctor may:

· Ask you questions about your current medical health insurance and symptoms.

· Do an eye exam.

·   Consider your blood pressure, execute a routine arteries test to be certain there is no serious loss of blood disorder.

Chapter 9

Eye Twitch

Nobody has discovered the reason for this yet, which a medical doctor might call blepharospasm. When it happens, your eyelid, usually the very best one, blinks, so you can't produce it end, sometimes it impacts both eyes. The lid moves every handful of seconds for a few momemts.

Doctors think maybe it's connected with:

·   Fatigue.

·   Stress.

·   Caffeine

Twitches are painless, harmless, and usually disappear completely independently. If the spasms are strong enough, they are able to cause your eyelids to shut and reopen totally. A lot of people possess eye spasms all day every day; they could continue for times, days, and even weeks.

It's rare, if a twitch doesn't disappear completely, it could make you wink or squint regularly.

Sometimes, the twitch can be viewed as an indicator of a lot more severe circumstances, like:

·   Blepharitis (inflamed eyelids).

·   Dry eyes.

·   Light sensitivity.

·   Pinkeye

Very rarely, it's an indicator of the mind or nerve disorder, such as for example:

·   Bell's palsy.

·   Dystonia.

·   Parkinson's disease.

·   Tourette's syndrome.

It could also be considered a side-effect of certain medications; the most typical consist of drugs that treat psychosis and epilepsy.

What exactly are the Types of Twitches?

You will see three common ones.

An eyelid twitch is often connected with life-style factors, like:

· Fatigue.

· Stress.

· Insomnia.

It could often be due to the constant using alcohol consumption, cigarettes, or caffeine. Additionally, it could be derived from the discomfort of the very best of the eyes (cornea) or the membranes that collect your eyelids (conjunctiva).

Benign essential blepharospasm usually arises in the centre to late adulthood and steadily gets worse. Record demonstrates in 12 months, only 2,000 people have problems with this ailment in the US. It isn't a substantial condition, but much more serious cases can hinder your way of life.

Causes include:

·   Fatigue.

·   Stress.

·   Bright light, wind flow or polluting of the surroundings.

It begins with nonstop blinking or vision irritation and gets worse until your eyes become delicate to light and get blurry and possess cosmetic spasms. In serious situations, the spasms could become so extreme that your eyelids stay shut for a number of hours.

Experts believe it results from a number of environmental and genetic factors; even though problem is normally arbitrary, it sometimes works in families.

A hemifacial spasm is rare; it entails both muscles round the mouth area plus your eyelid. Unlike the additional two types, it usually impacts only 1 area of the facial skin. Frequently, the reason is definitely an artery pressing around the facial nerve.

When should i see a doctor?

Make a meeting if:

·   The twitch is usually maintained to obtain additional when compared to a week.

·   Your eyelid closes completely.

·   Spasms involve other face muscles.

·   You observe inflammation, swelling, or release from an eye.

·   Your top eyelid drops

If a medical doctor suspects a brain or nerve problem reaches fault, she'll search for other common signs; she might mail you to a neurologist or various other specialist.

How can it be Treated?

Generally, a twitch will go away by itself; make sure you

get enough rest and cut back on alcohol consumption, cigarettes, and caffeine. If dry eye or irritated eye would be the cause, try over-the-counter artificial tears. That may often ease a twitch.

Doctors have still not found a finish to benign essential blepharospasm; however, several treatment plans make it less severe. The latest treatment is botulinum toxin (Botox, Dysport, Xeomin); additionally it is often found in combination having a hemifacial spasm.

Physician will inject small amounts into the vision muscles to greatly help ease the spasms; the effect lasts two months before it gradually wears off, and you'd need to carry out the procedure over again.

In moderate cases, a medical doctor might suggest medications like:

·   Clonazepam (Klonopin).

·   Lorazepam (Ativan).

·   Trihexyphenidyl hydrochloride (Artane, Trihexane, Tritane)

These usually provide just short-term alleviation.

Alternate treatments include:

- Biofeedback.

- Acupuncture.

- Hypnosis.

- Chiropractic.

- Nourishment therapy.

- Tinted glasses

Scientific tests haven't proven these treatments work.

If additional options fail, a medical doctor may suggest surgery; functioning called a myectomy, your physician will remove some of the muscles and nerves around your eyelid.

Surgery may also relieve the pressure from the artery on your own face nerve that creates a hemifacial spasm.

Acknowledgements

The Glory of this book success goes to God Almighty and my beautiful Family, Fans, Readers & well-wishers, Customers, and Friends for their endless support and encouragement.